Alzheimer's Ascent And Autumn's Alleviation

Providing compassionate and informative support to those struggling with Alzheimer's, empowering individuals and fostering hope

Rhysling Fitzwilliam

Contents

1 Understanding Alzheimer's

Alzheimer's disease, a progressive neurodegenerative disorder, gradually erodes cognitive functions, impacting memory, thinking, and behavior. Its insidious onset often makes early detection challenging. Initially, subtle memory lapses might be dismissed as normal age-related changes. However, as the disease progresses, these lapses become more frequent and pronounced, affecting daily life significantly. For instance, forgetting recent conversations, misplacing belongings repeatedly, or experiencing difficulty with familiar tasks are early warning signs requiring professional attention. The insidious nature of Alzheimer's emphasizes the importance of early detection and intervention to slow progression and maintain quality of life.

The diagnostic process for Alzheimer's involves a thorough neurological examination, cognitive testing, and often, brain imaging. Neuropsychological assessments, such as the Mini-Mental State Examination (MMSE), are crucial tools for evaluating cognitive abilities. These tests assess memory, orientation, language, and visuospatial skills.

Brain imaging techniques, including MRI and PET scans, help visualize brain structure and function, aiding in the differentiation between Alzheimer's and other conditions mimicking its symptoms. A comprehensive assessment is vital not only for diagnosis but also for tailoring an appropriate care plan. The process, while thorough, ultimately aims to provide a clear picture of the disease's stage and guide future management. This comprehensive approach is key to offering personalized and effective care.

Early diagnosis is pivotal for initiating timely interventions, maximizing the effectiveness of available therapies. Currently, no cure exists for Alzheimer's, but treatments can help manage symptoms and slow disease progression. Cholinesterase inhibitors and memantine are commonly prescribed medications that can help improve cognitive function and behavior in some individuals. However, their effectiveness varies depending on the stage of the disease and the individual's response. Beyond medication, non-pharmacological approaches, such as cognitive stimulation therapy and regular physical exercise, play a significant role in managing the disease's impact. These combined approaches represent a multifaceted approach to disease management, offering both medical and lifestyle interventions.

Moreover, lifestyle interventions are crucial for managing Alzheimer's and improving quality of life for both patients and their caregivers. Regular physical exercise has been shown to improve cognitive function, mood, and overall well-being. Engaging in activities that stimulate the brain, such as reading, puzzles, and social interaction, can also help maintain cognitive abilities. A healthy diet rich in fruits, vegetables, and omega-3 fatty acids is essential for overall health and may play a protective role against cognitive decline. Prioritizing sleep hygiene is vital, ensuring sufficient sleep to support brain function and overall health. These lifestyle modifications, alongside medication, form a holistic approach to managing Alzheimer's, enhancing quality of life.

Beyond the medical aspects, providing emotional support for patients and their families is equally crucial. Alzheimer's disease impacts not only the individual diagnosed but also the entire family unit. Caregivers often face significant emotional and physical burdens. Access to support groups, counseling services, and respite care can significantly alleviate stress and improve the caregiver's overall well-being. Understanding the emotional impact on families is vital for creating a comprehensive support system that addresses both the patient's and caregiver's needs. Open communication and mutual support are essential in navigating the challenges of living with Alzheimer's. Seeking professional assistance provides crucial resources for coping with the emotional tolls.

Finally, planning for the future is a necessary aspect of managing Alzheimer's disease. As the disease progresses, individuals may require increased levels of care, potentially necessitating long-term care facilities or home health services. Advance care planning, including discussions about end-of-life care wishes, is essential for ensuring that patients' preferences are respected. Financial planning is also important, considering the substantial costs associated with long-term care. Consulting with financial advisors and legal professionals can help families navigate these complex issues, ensuring they are prepared for the future. Proactive planning allows families to manage the logistical and financial implications of long-term care. This foresight empowers both the patient and their loved ones to navigate the future with greater confidence and peace of mind. Early planning for the future is crucial for minimizing stress and ensuring the best possible care.

1.1 Early Signs & Symptoms

Memory lapses are often the first noticeable sign, but they're subtle at first. Perhaps forgetting where you put your keys, or the name of a familiar acquaintance. These aren't necessarily cause for immediate alarm, as they happen to many people, but a consistent pattern of increasing forgetfulness should prompt further investigation. It might manifest as difficulty remembering recent events, while older memories remain intact, a peculiar disconnect that often goes unnoticed in the early stages. The person may also struggle to recall conversations or appointments, and retell stories repeatedly. This isn't about simple absentmindedness; it's a persistent struggle to retrieve information readily accessible in the past.

Beyond the obvious memory issues, changes in personality and behavior can emerge gradually. Once outgoing and engaging individuals might become withdrawn and isolated. What was once a vibrant social life shrinks as the individual loses interest in social activities. This isn't simply depression; it's a change in fundamental personality traits, a quiet fading of the person they once were. Increased irritability, apathy, or even aggression can appear, adding significant strain on family and caregivers. These behavioral changes often present as unexplained anxiety, frustration, or confusion, escalating unpredictably. The emotional landscape shifts, becoming less predictable, more challenging for both the patient and their loved ones. Understanding these nuances is key to providing compassionate support.

Difficulties with familiar tasks are another crucial indicator. Imagine someone struggling to prepare a meal they've made hundreds of times before, or getting lost in a neighborhood they've known for years. These aren't just moments of clumsiness; they represent a significant decline in cognitive function. The ability to perform everyday tasks, tasks once performed effortlessly, gradually erodes, leading to increased frustration and dependence. The individual might struggle with simple arithmetic or balancing a checkbook, tasks that previously required little thought. This progressive loss of functional abilities is a hallmark of Alzheimer's disease, highlighting the gradual encroachment of cognitive impairment on daily life. Recognizing these subtle shifts is critical for intervention.

Language impairments often appear as the disease progresses. Word-finding difficulties, struggling to name common objects, or speaking in incomplete sentences, these all signal a deterioration in cognitive processing. Conversations become more challenging, as the person struggles to articulate their thoughts and feelings. This doesn't mean a loss of intelligence; it's a manifestation of the disease's impact on brain function, affecting the ability to retrieve and organize language effectively. The difficulty in expressing oneself is deeply frustrating, underscoring the need for patience and understanding from those around them.

Spatial disorientation, a less discussed but equally important symptom, presents as difficulty navigating familiar spaces. Getting lost in one's own home, or misplacing objects repeatedly, suggests a decline in spatial reasoning and awareness. It's more than just forgetfulness; it's a loss of comprehension of one's surroundings. The individual may become disoriented in familiar environments, a frightening and discombobulating experience. This often requires careful assessment, as it can indicate not just cognitive decline but also a heightened risk of accidents.

Changes in judgment and decision-making are another key sign. Individuals might make impulsive or unusual decisions, exhibiting poor judgment in ways that were previously uncharacteristic. This can manifest as financial mismanagement, reckless driving, or inappropriate social behavior. These actions reflect a decline in executive function, the brain's ability to plan, organize, and execute tasks. It's crucial to recognize these changes, as they can have serious implications for the individual's safety and well-being. Intervention at this stage can help mitigate potential risks and protect the individual's interests. Family members should be vigilant and act promptly when such signs emerge. While these symptoms may appear individually, their combination paints a clearer picture. The key is to look for a pattern of increasing difficulties, a consistent decline in cognitive and functional abilities. It's about the trajectory of these changes, the gradual worsening of symptoms, not just an isolated incident. Early detection is crucial, as it allows for earlier intervention, potentially slowing the progression of the disease and improving the quality of life for both the patient and their caregivers. Don't hesitate to seek professional help if you notice these signs in yourself or a loved one. Early intervention can make a significant difference.

1.2 Diagnosis & Assessment

Reaching a definitive diagnosis of Alzheimer's disease can be a complex process, often requiring a multifaceted approach. It isn't a simple blood test; instead, it involves a careful evaluation of the individual's cognitive abilities, medical history, and neurological examination. This necessitates a collaborative effort between the patient, their family, and a team of healthcare professionals, potentially including neurologists, geriatricians, and psychologists. Remember, early detection is key to better management and slowing disease progression.

The diagnostic process typically begins with a thorough medical history, focusing on the onset and progression of symptoms. This includes detailed questioning about memory problems, changes in personality or behavior, difficulty with language or problem-solving, and any other cognitive difficulties. Family members play a vital role in providing information about the patient's cognitive decline, as they often observe subtle changes that the individual themselves might not notice. Detailed accounts of the patient's daily functioning are essential, such as whether they can manage their finances, prepare meals, or navigate familiar locations.

Neuropsychological testing forms a cornerstone of the assessment. These tests assess various cognitive domains, including memory, attention, language, executive function, and visuospatial abilities. The results provide a quantitative measure of the individual's cognitive performance, compared to age-matched norms. Scores on these tests help pinpoint specific cognitive deficits and track their progression over time. It's crucial to understand that these are not pass/fail tests, but rather tools that provide valuable insights into the nature and severity of cognitive impairment.

Beyond cognitive testing, a comprehensive neurological examination is crucial. This examination evaluates the patient's reflexes, coordination, gait, and other neurological functions. The goal is to rule out other neurological conditions that might mimic Alzheimer's symptoms, such as stroke, Parkinson's disease, or other forms of dementia. Brain imaging techniques, such as magnetic resonance imaging (MRI) or computed tomography (CT) scans, are often employed to visualize the brain's structure, helping to identify any abnormalities such as strokes, tumors, or significant brain atrophy.

However, even with these advanced techniques, a definitive diagnosis of Alzheimer's disease often relies on a process of exclusion. Other potential causes of cognitive impairment need to be ruled out before a diagnosis can be confidently made. This highlights the importance of a multidisciplinary approach, bringing together specialists who can offer different perspectives and diagnostic insights. The team will collaborate to interpret the results of various tests and examinations, weighing all the information before coming to a conclusive diagnosis.

Furthermore, it's crucial to recognize that the diagnostic process can be emotionally challenging for both the patient and their family. The uncertainty surrounding the diagnosis and the potential impact on the individual's future can cause considerable anxiety and fear. Open and honest communication between healthcare professionals and the patient's support system is paramount to alleviate concerns and provide emotional support throughout the process. Providing education and resources about Alzheimer's disease helps alleviate misunderstandings and fosters a sense of empowerment. Understanding the diagnostic process and its limitations helps manage expectations and prepares everyone for the challenges ahead. The aim is to navigate this complex journey with compassion, providing support and ensuring that the patient and their loved ones feel understood and supported. Remember, a prompt and accurate diagnosis lays the foundation for appropriate management and intervention, helping to improve the quality of life for the individual and their family.

2 Coping Strategies for Patients

Maintaining a sense of normalcy is crucial. Even small, familiar routines can provide comfort and a sense of security. Encourage participation in activities the person enjoyed before the diagnosis, adapting them as needed to accommodate their current abilities. A simple walk in the park, listening to favorite music, or looking at old photographs can trigger positive memories and emotions. Remember, it's about finding joy in the present, even if it's a modified version of what it once was. Small victories, like successfully brushing teeth or completing a simple puzzle, should be celebrated and acknowledged. This positive reinforcement helps to maintain self-esteem and a sense of accomplishment.

For those experiencing memory loss, visual aids and reminders can be incredibly helpful. Large, clear calendars, labeled containers for belongings, and strategically placed notes can provide important cues. Consider using photo albums or memory boxes filled with cherished items to stimulate recall and conversation. Remember to speak clearly and slowly, using simple language. Avoid overwhelming them with too much information at once. Patience is key. It's often not about correcting their mistakes, but acknowledging their feelings and validating their experiences.

Maintaining a sense of independence is paramount to preserving dignity. Offer choices whenever possible, allowing the individual to feel a sense of control over their life. This could be as simple as choosing between two different outfits or deciding what to have for lunch. Even small choices can make a significant difference in their emotional well-being. Encourage self-care activities, such as bathing or dressing, to the extent they are able. Provide assistance only when necessary, avoiding unnecessary dependence. It's a delicate balance between supporting them and allowing them to retain their autonomy. Celebrate their successes, no matter how small, and offer encouragement during moments of frustration or confusion.

Creating a safe and supportive environment is essential. This involves removing potential hazards from the home, such as loose rugs or unsecured electrical cords. Establishing clear and consistent routines reduces confusion and anxiety. A predictable daily schedule provides structure and helps the person anticipate what will happen next, minimizing uncertainty. Consistent caregivers are ideal; familiar faces provide comfort and reduce stress. Simple routines like mealtimes and bedtimes can become anchors for the person living with Alzheimer's. Try to make the environment calming and soothing by using soft colors, calming music, and comfortable furniture.

Cognitive stimulation is important, but it needs to be tailored to the individual's abilities. Don't force activities; instead, observe what they enjoy and adapt activities to suit their current cognitive function. Engaging in simple crafts, listening to music, or reminiscing over photographs can provide valuable cognitive stimulation without being overwhelming. The focus should be on pleasure and engagement, not performance. Puzzles, coloring books, and large-print books can be beneficial, and don't underestimate the power of simple conversation. Share stories and memories; reminiscing can help strengthen connections and evoke positive emotions.

Adapting routines to the progression of the disease is vital. As the disease progresses, routines and activities may need to be modified or simplified. It's crucial to remain flexible and adapt to the changing needs of the person with Alzheimer's. This might involve breaking down complex tasks into smaller, more manageable steps, offering assistance as needed, and being prepared for unexpected changes in behavior or mood. The goal remains to maintain as much quality of life and independence as possible. This adaptable approach will allow you to cope with the changing landscape of the disease effectively.

Remember, there will be days when it feels overwhelming. Don't hesitate to seek support from family, friends, or professional caregivers. Utilizing respite care can provide valuable time for self-care and prevent caregiver burnout. This time away isn't a sign of failure, but rather a sign of self-preservation. It's crucial to remember to take care of yourself so that you can continue to provide the best possible care for your loved one. Remember to celebrate the small victories and cherish the moments you share.

Focus on building positive relationships and fostering a sense of connection. Even when communication becomes challenging, non-verbal cues such as touch, smiles, and expressions of affection can still convey love and support. Spend quality time together, engaging in activities that both of you enjoy. The goal is to create a sense of peace, security, and connection, even as the disease progresses. Maintaining these positive relationships is an essential part of maintaining dignity and fostering hope. Remember that love and connection can transcend verbal communication.

2.1 Daily Life Management

Maintaining a consistent daily routine is crucial. The predictability reduces anxiety and confusion, providing a sense of security and normalcy for someone with Alzheimer's. Simple, visual schedules, perhaps using photographs or icons, can be incredibly helpful. Think about incorporating familiar activities they enjoy, even if they only remember parts of them; the emotional connection is vital. Break down complex tasks into smaller, manageable steps. Instead of saying "Get ready for bed," try a series of prompts: "It's time for your pajamas," then "Let's brush your teeth," and finally "Time for bed now." Consistency in these steps, repeated daily, creates a comforting ritual. Remember, patience is key; unexpected reactions are common, and gentle redirection is more effective than forceful correction.

For eating, establish regular mealtimes and create a calm, distraction-free environment. Familiar foods, presented attractively, often encourage better intake. If swallowing becomes difficult, consider pureed foods or softer textures. Never pressure someone to eat; it only increases stress. Observe their eating habits closely, noting any changes in appetite or preference, and report these to their physician. Small, frequent meals might be better tolerated than three large ones. Consider offering healthy snacks between meals to maintain energy levels throughout the day. Remember always to consult their doctor or a registered dietician for dietary advice tailored to their specific needs and health status. Their guidance is paramount to ensure adequate nutrition, particularly if they have any coexisting conditions.

Personal hygiene can become challenging. Maintaining a routine is important, but remember flexibility is equally so. Adapt the routine to their level of comprehension and ability. A supportive and patient approach is essential. Encourage participation as much as possible, even if it's just a small part of the process. Using gentle reminders and positive reinforcement fosters cooperation. Consider using adaptive tools designed to assist with bathing or dressing, making the process easier and less frustrating for both the individual and the caregiver. If assistance is needed, ensure privacy and respect their dignity throughout the process. Always prioritize safety; consider non-slip mats in the shower and grab bars for added security. Never rush the process; allow ample time, ensuring comfort and reducing stress.

Dressing can be simplified with loose clothing, easy-to-fasten garments, or even elastic-waist clothing. Lay out the clothes in the order they should be put on, using pictures as visual aids if helpful. Keep the clothes readily accessible, organizing them in a way that is easily understandable. Consider pre-selecting outfits for the week to reduce decision-making stress. If someone resists getting dressed, don't force it; try again later. If the weather changes drastically, immediately adjust the clothing to ensure their comfort. Adapt to their preferences and work within their capabilities, adjusting as their needs change.

Physical activity remains important; even gentle exercises improve mood and well-being. Simple activities such as walking, chair exercises, or even just moving their arms and legs can make a difference. Always consult their physician before starting any exercise program to ensure it's suitable for their physical condition. Incorporate activities they enjoy, such as gardening, dancing, or playing with pets. Music therapy can also be incredibly beneficial, improving mood and memory recall. Engage them in activities that stimulate their senses and provide enjoyment. Remember to tailor the activity to their current capabilities, focusing on safety and preventing falls. Regular movement prevents stiffness and promotes a sense of well-being, positively impacting overall quality of life.

Sleep disturbances are common. Establishing a regular sleep schedule and creating a relaxing bedtime routine is beneficial. Ensure their bedroom is dark, quiet, and comfortable. Avoid caffeine and alcohol before bedtime. A warm bath or a gentle massage can promote relaxation. If they have difficulty falling asleep, consult their doctor to rule out any underlying medical conditions that may be contributing to the sleep disruption. Avoid overstimulating activities before bed, and create a calm and peaceful environment conducive to sleep. Maintaining a consistent sleep schedule, even on weekends, will significantly improve their sleep quality. Regular daytime activity also helps regulate their sleep-wake cycle.

Social interaction remains crucial. Engage them in conversations about familiar topics, sharing happy memories and using simple language. Include them in family activities, even if their participation is limited. Their presence adds value to the event. Regular visits from family and friends offer vital social stimulation. If they become withdrawn, gently encourage interaction but avoid forcing it. Support groups for caregivers and individuals with Alzheimer's provide vital emotional support and a sense of community. Their shared experiences and insights can make an immeasurable difference. Encourage interaction through simple, joyful activities, focusing on building positive emotional connections.

2.2 Memory Aids & Techniques

Utilizing memory aids and techniques can significantly improve the quality of life for individuals with Alzheimer's disease. These tools aren't about curing the disease, but rather about maximizing cognitive function and independence for as long as possible. Remember, small, consistent efforts often yield the best results. Patience is crucial; introducing new techniques gradually is more effective than overwhelming the individual.

For example, consider using visual aids. Photographs, calendars with large, clear print, and color-coded labels can assist with orientation and daily tasks. A picture of a toothbrush can remind someone to brush their teeth; similarly, a photo of a loved one might spark a meaningful conversation, even when verbal recall is limited. Moreover, these visual cues offer a sense of familiarity and security in a potentially confusing world. The goal is not to replace memory, but to provide supportive scaffolding.

Furthermore, environmental adaptations play a significant role. A clutter-free environment reduces confusion and promotes a sense of calm. Clearly labeled drawers and cabinets make it easier to locate personal items, reducing frustration and anxiety. Establish consistent routines for daily activities such as eating, bathing, and sleeping. Predictability reduces the cognitive load and fosters a sense of security. Even small, consistent changes in the environment can make a noticeable difference in reducing stress and improving engagement.

Engaging in reminiscence therapy, a structured method of recalling past memories, is another powerful technique. Sharing old photographs, listening to familiar music, or discussing cherished memories can stimulate cognitive function and evoke positive emotions. These sessions are not just about recollection; they're about connecting with the individual on an emotional level, reinforcing their sense of self and identity. These memories, even if fragmented, retain their power to enrich the present moment.

Structured activities, such as puzzles, simple games, or crafts, can help maintain cognitive stimulation. Choose activities that are appropriate for the individual's current abilities, gradually increasing the level of difficulty as they progress. Focus on activities they find enjoyable, rather than imposing tasks that feel overwhelming. Remember, the emphasis is on engagement and enjoyment, not on achieving perfect results. The benefits extend beyond cognitive stimulation to encompass emotional well-being.

Utilizing external memory aids such as notebooks, calendars, or digital reminders can provide a helpful support system. Keep these aids visible and easily accessible. Remember to keep entries simple and clear, utilizing large print and visual cues when possible. The key is to make it easy to use and understand. The aim is to enhance, not replace, the person's inherent memory abilities. Technology, too, has a role to play, but only as a supplement to simpler methods.

Verbal cues and reminders can also be effective, but must be used with sensitivity and understanding. Avoid patronizing language or correcting the individual repeatedly. Instead, offer gentle guidance and encouragement. A simple, reassuring tone and patience are vital aspects of any strategy. Consistency in communication and approach is as valuable as the method itself.

Creating a memory book or scrapbook, filled with photos, mementos, and significant events, can be a rewarding project. Involve the individual in the process as much as possible, fostering a sense of participation and ownership. This is more than just a memory aid; it's a tangible representation of their life and identity. The act of creating it is often as beneficial as its subsequent use.

Finally, remember that caregiver well-being is crucial. Caregivers need to prioritize their own health and seek support when needed. There are resources available, such as support groups and respite care, which can provide much-needed assistance and relief. The journey of caring for someone with Alzheimer's is a marathon, not a sprint. Sustaining your own well-being ensures you can provide the best possible care for your loved one. Prioritize self-care; you cannot pour from an empty cup.

2.3 Maintaining Dignity & Independence

Preserving a sense of self-worth and autonomy is paramount for individuals navigating the challenges of Alzheimer's disease. It's not about denying the disease's presence; it's about finding ways to nurture their remaining capabilities and celebrate their unique identity, even as cognitive abilities decline. This involves a multifaceted approach, encompassing both practical adaptations and a shift in mindset from caregivers and loved ones alike.

For the individual with Alzheimer's, maintaining a sense of control, however small, can significantly impact their emotional well-being. Encourage their participation in daily routines, even if it's just choosing their outfit for the day or helping with simple tasks like folding laundry. These seemingly insignificant choices foster a sense of agency, a powerful antidote to the feelings of helplessness that can accompany cognitive decline. Remember, it's about adapting, not abandoning, their involvement.

Caregivers often struggle with the shift in roles. The person they knew, independent and capable, is gradually changing. This transition requires immense patience and a willingness to adjust expectations. Instead of focusing on what they can no longer do, concentrate on what they can still accomplish, however small the task. Celebrate those achievements, however modest. Acknowledge their efforts and provide positive reinforcement. This fosters a sense of worth and minimizes feelings of frustration for both the individual and the caregiver.

Adaptations to the home environment can also play a critical role. Simple changes, such as clear signage for frequently used rooms or strategically placed items, can reduce confusion and enhance independence. Consider using visual cues rather than verbal instructions, as visual memory often remains longer than verbal memory. Create a calming and predictable routine to minimize stress and anxiety—a consistent schedule provides a sense of order and security in a world that may feel increasingly unpredictable. Remember, consistency is key in minimizing confusion and maintaining a sense of stability for the individual.

Maintaining social connections is equally vital. Even in the later stages, meaningful interactions can bring joy and stimulation. Encourage visits from loved ones, engaging in activities they enjoyed prior to diagnosis, even if it's just listening to their favorite music or looking at old photographs. These shared moments provide comfort and validation, preserving their sense of connection to the world and the people they cherish. Organize activities and engage them in ways that are meaningful and enjoyable; it's crucial to cater to their current abilities and interests.

Respecting their dignity is paramount throughout the entire journey. Avoid patronizing language or infantilizing behavior. Address them respectfully, acknowledging their feelings and experiences. Treat them as individuals with their own thoughts, feelings, and history, not merely as a diagnosis. Active listening and empathetic responses are crucial. Even when communication becomes challenging, nonverbal communication, such as a gentle touch or a warm smile, can convey empathy and understanding, maintaining a connection on a deeper level.

The importance of creating a safe and secure environment cannot be overstated. This isn't just about physical safety; it's about creating an environment that supports their emotional and psychological well-being. Reduce potential hazards within the home, creating a space where they can move freely and confidently. This contributes to their overall sense of security and independence, allowing them to retain a degree of control over their surroundings. Making sure to remove anything that might trigger falls or confusion is essential.

Finally, remember that maintaining dignity and independence is an ongoing process, requiring constant adaptation and flexibility. There will be good days and bad days. The key is to focus on the small victories, celebrating the successes and adapting strategies when needed. The journey is complex, but preserving their dignity and enabling their independence is achievable with patience, understanding, and tailored support. It is an act of compassion and love that profoundly impacts the quality of life for both the individual and their caregivers, fostering a more hopeful and enriching experience. This is not just about managing the disease; it's about honoring the person living with it.

3 Caregiver Support & Resources

The emotional toll on caregivers is immense. Feelings of isolation, exhaustion, and grief are common, and it's crucial to acknowledge these feelings as valid. Seeking professional support, whether through therapy, counseling, or support groups, is not a sign of weakness but a testament to your strength and commitment. Remember to prioritize self-care, even in small ways: taking a walk, reading a book, or simply enjoying a quiet moment can make a significant difference. Building a strong support network of friends, family, or fellow caregivers is vital. Sharing your experiences and connecting with others who understand can alleviate feelings of loneliness and provide invaluable emotional support. Don't hesitate to ask for help; your well-being is just as important as the care you provide.

Practical assistance is often the most immediate need for caregivers. Respite care, which provides temporary relief from caregiving responsibilities, is invaluable. It allows you to recharge and return to your caregiving role with renewed energy. Explore in-home care services, which can provide assistance with tasks like bathing, dressing, and meal preparation. Adult day care centers offer structured programs that provide stimulation and social interaction for the person with Alzheimer's while giving you a much-needed break. Caregiver training programs offer valuable education and support, equipping you with the skills and knowledge to manage the challenges of Alzheimer's more effectively. They teach techniques for managing behaviors, communication strategies, and safety measures.

Financial planning is an often-overlooked yet critical aspect of Alzheimer's care. The costs associated with medical care, medications, and in-home assistance can be substantial. It's essential to review your insurance coverage, explore long-term care insurance options, and understand the financial resources available to you. Consult with a financial advisor specializing in elder care to create a comprehensive financial plan that ensures both your and your loved one's financial security. Investigate government assistance programs, such as Medicaid and Medicare, to determine your eligibility for financial aid. Planning early and understanding available resources will significantly lessen the financial burden associated with long-term care.

Your community offers a wealth of resources to support you in your caregiving journey. Local senior centers often provide social activities, transportation services, and educational programs for both caregivers and individuals with Alzheimer's. Religious organizations often offer support groups and spiritual guidance. Alzheimer's associations provide vital information, support groups, and educational resources tailored to the needs of caregivers. They frequently organize workshops, seminars, and online forums where caregivers can share experiences and learn new skills. Don't underestimate the power of these community resources; they can become a lifeline, providing support, information, and connection.

Legal considerations are crucial, particularly as the disease progresses. You should consider establishing a power of attorney for healthcare and finances. This ensures that your loved one's wishes are respected regarding medical decisions and financial matters. A will should be updated to reflect the changing circumstances. Consult with an estate planning attorney to understand the legal ramifications of Alzheimer's and to prepare for potential future scenarios. They can guide you through the process of creating legally sound documents that protect your loved one's interests and provide you with the legal framework necessary to manage their care. Don't delay this crucial step; early planning ensures smooth transitions and reduces future stress and uncertainty.

3.1 Emotional Well-being

Caring for someone with Alzheimer's is a marathon, not a sprint, and emotional well-being for the caregiver is just as crucial as the patient's physical health. Neglecting your own emotional health jeopardizes your ability to provide effective care. Remember, you are not alone in this journey. Many resources exist to help you navigate this emotionally demanding path.

Burnout is a real threat. The relentless demands of caregiving can lead to exhaustion, both physically and emotionally. Symptoms can range from irritability and impatience to feelings of hopelessness and despair. Recognizing these signs early is vital. Actively prioritizing self-care isn't selfish; it's essential for your sustainability. This allows you to continue offering the best possible care to your loved one without compromising your well-being.

Building a support system is paramount. Lean on friends, family, support groups, or even professional therapists. Sharing your burdens with others reduces the weight you carry alone. Don't hesitate to ask for help. People genuinely want to support you, but they might not know how unless you tell them. This support system shouldn't be underestimated. It offers emotional sustenance during challenging times, enabling you to withstand the emotional toll of caregiving.

Finding moments of respite is critical for preventing burnout. Arrange for respite care, even if it's just for a few hours a week. This allows you to recharge, engage in activities you enjoy, and return to caregiving with renewed energy and perspective. Scheduling regular breaks isn't a luxury; it's a necessity, a vital component in your ongoing caregiving journey. These breaks maintain your ability to provide attentive care.

Engage in activities you find enjoyable and relaxing. This could be anything from reading a book to taking a walk in nature, or even simply enjoying a quiet cup of tea. These activities provide much-needed emotional replenishment, helping you cope with the stress of caregiving. Prioritizing these activities, even for short periods, improves your mental resilience and emotional stability. It's a key strategy to ensure long-term caregiving success.

Consider professional help if needed. A therapist can provide a safe space to process your emotions, develop coping strategies, and learn techniques for managing stress. Don't feel ashamed to seek professional assistance. It's a sign of strength, not weakness. Accessing professional support is a proactive step towards maintaining your emotional stability. Many therapists specialize in supporting caregivers of individuals with Alzheimer's and dementia.

Maintain healthy lifestyle habits. Adequate sleep, nutritious food, and regular exercise are crucial for both physical and emotional well-being. These habits aren't just beneficial for your physical health; they're crucial in enhancing your ability to cope with emotional stress. These practices directly impact your emotional resilience, increasing your capacity to provide quality care.

Remember that feelings of grief, anger, or sadness are normal. Allow yourself to feel these emotions without judgment. Suppressing them only intensifies their impact. Understanding that these feelings are natural reactions to the circumstances provides validation and helps you cope in a healthier way. It's important to acknowledge and process these emotions constructively.

Celebrate the small victories and cherish the moments you have with your loved one. Focusing on the positive aspects of your relationship helps maintain emotional balance and perspective. It is a crucial factor in sustaining emotional strength and resilience during challenging times. Focusing on shared experiences and memories nourishes your connection despite the disease's challenges.

Accept that you cannot control the disease's progression, but you can control your response to it. Focusing on what you can control—your own well-being, the quality of care you provide, and your emotional response—empowers you and reduces feelings of helplessness. This approach allows for a more constructive and positive focus during a difficult time. It offers a pathway to resilience and strength in caregiving. You may not be able to change the disease, but you can change how you respond to it. This shift in focus impacts your emotional state significantly, impacting your capacity for effective caregiving.

Ultimately, prioritizing your emotional well-being is not a luxury; it is a necessity. By actively engaging in self-care, building a support system, and seeking professional help when needed, you can navigate this challenging journey with greater resilience and strength. You are essential in the caregiving process, and taking care of yourself ensures you can continue to provide the best possible care for your loved one, extending the time and quality of moments shared. Remember to cherish those moments.

3.2 Practical Assistance

The daily grind of caring for someone with Alzheimer's can feel overwhelming, a constant barrage of needs and anxieties. You're not alone. Many caregivers find themselves struggling to juggle medications, appointments, and the emotional toll of witnessing a loved one's decline. Remember to prioritize your own well-being; it's not selfish, it's essential. Taking breaks, even short ones, can make a huge difference in preventing burnout. Consider engaging in activities you enjoy, even if it's just for fifteen minutes a day. This could be reading, listening to music, or simply enjoying a cup of tea in quiet contemplation. These small acts of self-care will replenish your emotional reserves, enabling you to provide better care.

Respite care is a valuable resource frequently overlooked. This involves utilizing temporary care services, allowing you a much-needed break.

These services can range from a few hours to several days, offering a vital opportunity to recharge and prevent caregiver burnout. Investigate local organizations and agencies; many offer subsidized or free respite care options, lessening the financial burden. Remember, seeking support isn't a sign of weakness; it's a demonstration of strength and responsible caregiving. Don't hesitate to accept help when offered, and don't be afraid to ask for it when you need it.

Organizing your loved one's medications can be a significant challenge. A medication organizer, a simple pill dispenser with daily compartments, can greatly simplify the process, reducing stress and the risk of medication errors. Working closely with the doctor and pharmacist to ensure the correct dosage and timing is crucial. Understanding the potential side effects of each medication is equally vital, enabling you to promptly identify and address any issues. Maintaining a clear and concise record of all medications, including dosages and administration times, is invaluable, facilitating easier communication with medical professionals. It also provides a readily available reference should any questions arise.

Maintaining a structured daily routine can be incredibly helpful for individuals with Alzheimer's. Consistency offers a sense of stability and predictability, reducing confusion and anxiety. Simple visual aids, such as schedules or checklists, can assist in guiding daily activities. These aids provide a clear and concise roadmap to the day's events, helping to manage transitions more effectively. Incorporate familiar activities into the routine; this could involve listening to favorite music, engaging in gentle exercise, or spending time in a familiar environment. Remember to break down complex tasks into smaller, manageable steps to avoid overwhelming your loved one.

Safety is paramount. Home modifications are often necessary to ensure a safe living environment. Removing tripping hazards, installing grab bars in the bathroom, and ensuring good lighting are essential precautions. Consider installing a medical alert system, providing immediate access to emergency services if needed. This can offer considerable peace of mind, knowing that help is readily available in case of an accident or emergency. Regular safety checks are equally vital, identifying and addressing any potential hazards before they become a problem. Remember, a safe environment fosters independence and reduces the risk of injury.

Connecting with other caregivers can provide invaluable support. Support groups offer a safe space to share experiences, exchange advice, and simply vent frustrations. These groups provide a sense of community, reminding you that you're not alone in your journey. Participating in a support group can alleviate feelings of isolation and overwhelm, providing renewed energy and perspective. Sharing stories and learning from others' experiences can offer practical solutions and emotional comfort. Online forums and communities also offer an additional avenue for connection and support, expanding your reach and providing a broader range of perspectives. Don't underestimate the power of shared experiences and mutual support.

Remember, caring for someone with Alzheimer's is a marathon, not a sprint. Pace yourself, seek support, and remember to celebrate the small victories along the way. Every act of compassion, every moment of connection, makes a difference. Your dedication and love are invaluable.

3.3 Financial Planning

Facing the financial realities of Alzheimer's can feel overwhelming. The disease's progression often necessitates significant changes in lifestyle, care arrangements, and expenses, creating considerable financial strain on both the individual with Alzheimer's and their family. Early planning is crucial to mitigate these challenges and ensure financial security. It's not just about money; it's about protecting your loved one's quality of life and securing your own peace of mind during a difficult time.

Understanding the costs associated with Alzheimer's care is the first step. These costs are variable and depend on several factors, including the stage of the disease, the level of care required, and the availability of support services in your area. Home care, assisted living, and nursing home care all carry different price tags, significantly impacting your overall budget. Consider the potential need for specialized medical equipment, therapies, and medications. Additionally, factor in potential loss of income for the caregiver who may need to reduce work hours or quit their job entirely. This holistic approach to financial assessment is essential to accurate planning.

Legal and financial professionals can offer invaluable guidance. Consulting an elder law attorney is highly recommended. They can help navigate the complexities of Medicaid, Medicare, and long-term care insurance, ensuring you understand your options and entitlements. These specialists possess the knowledge to devise a plan that best protects your assets while securing appropriate care for your loved one. Don't hesitate to seek their expertise; their guidance can prevent significant financial pitfalls later on. They can also assist in establishing durable power of attorney and healthcare proxies, crucial legal documents granting another individual the authority to make financial and healthcare decisions on behalf of the person with Alzheimer's if they become incapacitated.

Long-term care insurance is a crucial consideration for financial planning. While the premiums can be substantial, the protection it offers against the potentially devastating costs of long-term care is considerable. Assess the potential benefits relative to the premiums to determine its suitability for your circumstances. Understanding the policy's terms, coverage limits, and waiting periods is vital before committing. Early purchasing is typically more advantageous, offering lower premiums and broader coverage options. Exploring different policy options and comparing providers is also advised to secure the most beneficial arrangement.

Beyond insurance, explore available government assistance programs. Medicaid and Medicare can provide significant financial relief, but eligibility criteria vary widely depending on your location and individual circumstances. Research your local and state programs thoroughly to identify any benefits your family might qualify for. This may include home health aide services, adult day care programs, or respite care for caregivers, all of which can significantly reduce the financial burden. Be proactive in gathering necessary documentation to simplify the application process and ensure a timely approval.

Retirement planning also takes on added significance in the face of Alzheimer's. The costs associated with long-term care can severely deplete retirement savings. Consider adjusting your retirement savings strategy to account for potential Alzheimer's-related expenses. If retirement is imminent, assess your current savings and anticipate the potential impact of ongoing care costs. This may involve working longer, delaying retirement, or reducing your planned lifestyle expenses. Financial planning should always be adaptable and flexible, so adjust accordingly.

Open communication within the family is paramount. Honest conversations about financial resources, expectations, and potential future needs can prevent misunderstandings and alleviate stress. Sharing information and establishing clear roles and responsibilities will ensure everyone understands their contribution to the overall care plan. Regular family meetings can facilitate effective communication and ensure adjustments can be made as needed. Such transparency can build a strong support system during a challenging period.

Finally, remember that seeking professional financial advice is not a sign of weakness; it is a sign of proactive planning. Financial advisors can help create a personalized budget, evaluate financial risk, and develop strategies for managing the financial implications of Alzheimer's. They can offer objective counsel and provide guidance tailored to your specific needs and circumstances, ensuring that your family's financial well-being is secured, enabling you to focus on providing compassionate care. Don't underestimate the value of this support; it is an investment in your future and your loved one's well-being.

3.4 Community Support

Harnessing the power of community support is vital for navigating the challenges of Alzheimer's. It's not just about practical assistance; it's about building a web of understanding and empathy that surrounds both the individual with Alzheimer's and their caregivers. This network can significantly lessen the burden and offer a sense of belonging often lost amidst the disease's progression. Remember, you're not alone in this journey.

Local support groups offer an invaluable lifeline. These groups provide a safe space for sharing experiences, anxieties, and triumphs. Connecting with others facing similar challenges creates a sense of community, reducing feelings of isolation and fostering mutual understanding. The opportunity to share practical tips, coping mechanisms, and even just a listening ear can prove incredibly beneficial. Many groups offer educational sessions and guest speakers, further enhancing their value. Don't hesitate to explore local senior centers, hospitals, or Alzheimer's associations for information on these groups near you.

Beyond formal support groups, consider the informal networks around you. Friends, family members, neighbors, and even faith communities can offer invaluable support in various ways. Friends might offer respite care, allowing caregivers a much-needed break. Family could assist with errands, meal preparation, or financial management. Neighbors can offer a friendly check-in, offering a simple but significant connection. Your faith community, if applicable, may have resources and support networks specifically tailored to individuals with Alzheimer's and their families. Leveraging these existing relationships strengthens the overall support system.

Utilizing community resources extends beyond personal connections. Many communities offer specialized services designed to help people with Alzheimer's and their caregivers. These could include adult day care centers providing structured activities and social interaction, respite care services for temporary relief, home healthcare agencies offering assistance with personal care and medical needs, and transportation services facilitating access to appointments and social events. A thorough investigation into your local resources is crucial. Contact your local health department, area agency on aging, or Alzheimer's Association for details on the availability and access to such programs. Proactive research will significantly enhance your access to support.

Furthermore, consider exploring volunteer opportunities. Participating in programs related to Alzheimer's care can provide a rewarding experience, fostering a deeper understanding of the challenges faced by those with the disease and their families. Volunteering often connects you with valuable resources and expands your network of support. This is not just beneficial for the community; it can be personally enriching for the caregiver, reducing stress and fostering a sense of purpose. Contact local charities, hospitals, or senior centers to inquire about available volunteer positions. Remember, volunteering offers a chance to give back, and the benefits extend beyond the recipient.

Finally, building a proactive support network requires communication. Openly communicating your needs and challenges to your loved ones and community will encourage others to offer help. Don't feel embarrassed to ask for assistance. Most people want to help, but they may not know how. Clear communication ensures you receive the support you need when you need it most. Creating a detailed care plan that outlines specific needs and preferences is also helpful, ensuring clear and consistent support. Remember, acceptance of help is not a sign of weakness, but a testament to your strength and recognition of the importance of community in navigating this journey. This proactive approach allows for effective support mechanisms to be built around both the individual with Alzheimer's and those caring for them. The more interconnected the network, the better equipped everyone will be to face the challenges ahead.

3.5 Legal Considerations

Navigating the complex legal landscape surrounding Alzheimer's disease is crucial for both patients and their caregivers. Early planning can significantly alleviate future burdens and protect the rights and well-being of the affected individual. One of the most important initial steps involves creating a comprehensive power of attorney for healthcare decisions. This legal document designates a trusted individual to make medical choices on behalf of the patient when they are no longer capable of doing so themselves. Choosing the right person, someone you completely trust with your well-being, is absolutely vital and should be a carefully considered decision. This person will need to understand your wishes, preferences, and values regarding healthcare.

Understanding the nuances of healthcare directives is paramount.

These legally binding documents outline your preferences for medical treatment, particularly in end-of-life situations. A well-drafted healthcare directive ensures your wishes are respected, even if you are unable to communicate them directly. It's advisable to discuss your preferences openly with your chosen healthcare agent, ensuring they fully grasp your intentions. Reviewing and updating these documents regularly, especially as the disease progresses, is essential to reflect any changes in your circumstances or wishes. Remember, these documents aren't set in stone; life, and illness, can be unpredictable. Adaptability in planning is key.

Beyond healthcare decisions, financial planning takes on immense significance. Establishing a durable power of attorney for finances allows a designated person to manage your financial affairs if you become incapacitated. This includes paying bills, managing investments, and accessing funds for your care. This process requires careful consideration of who will assume this responsibility; you need someone reliable, organized, and capable of handling financial matters. Open communication with this person about your financial situation and your wishes regarding its management is crucial to avoid future conflicts and misunderstandings. This person needs full transparency to ensure the effective management of your funds. Regular review is equally important in this area; ensuring finances are effectively and legally managed is an ongoing process.

Estate planning becomes increasingly important as Alzheimer's progresses. A will designates how your assets will be distributed after your passing. This ensures your wishes regarding the inheritance of your property are adhered to. Without a will, the distribution of your assets is determined by state law, which may not align with your intentions. This is particularly crucial if you have significant assets, or complex family dynamics. Careful consideration and planning in this area prevent considerable legal and emotional distress for your loved ones, reducing potential disputes and conflict among family members. Finally, understanding the implications of long-term care insurance is crucial. As Alzheimer's disease progresses, the need for long-term care, often requiring considerable financial resources, is likely. Long-term care insurance can help alleviate the financial burden associated with this care, assisting in funding various levels of care, from assisted living facilities to in-home care. This insurance policy is often purchased much earlier in life, when you're healthier and premiums are generally more affordable. However, if you do not already have this insurance, it's advisable to explore Medicaid and Medicare coverage options and fully understand the process of applying for and qualifying for these beneficial programs. Navigating this complex area of healthcare funding can be challenging, and consulting with legal and financial professionals is highly recommended.

4 Communication & Interaction

Maintaining clear and consistent communication is paramount when caring for someone with Alzheimer's. Simple, direct sentences are often most effective. Avoid complex instructions or abstract concepts. Instead of asking, "What would you like to wear today?", try presenting two options: "Would you prefer the blue shirt or the red shirt?" This focused approach minimizes confusion and frustration for the individual. Remember, patience is key; rushing will only increase anxiety. Repeating yourself calmly is acceptable, even expected. Don't take their reactions personally; they're not intentionally being difficult. Your unwavering patience and understanding will build a stronger bond.

For many caregivers, nonverbal communication becomes incredibly significant. A gentle touch, a warm smile, or a reassuring presence can often convey more than words. Observe their body language—a furrowed brow, clenched fists, or restless movements might indicate discomfort or distress, even if they can't verbally express it. Responding to these subtle cues with empathy and appropriate action is crucial for maintaining a peaceful and supportive environment. Remember the power of a simple, loving gesture.

Building positive relationships goes beyond just practical communication. Engage in activities they enjoy. Perhaps reminiscing over old photos, listening to familiar music, or gently engaging in a simple, repetitive task. These shared experiences create moments of connection and joy. Remember cherished memories, and share stories with them, even if they don't fully recall the details. Your presence and engagement offer a sense of comfort and familiarity, fostering a sense of security and belonging. The goal isn't necessarily to recall specific events but to share the emotional connection.

Consider the environment's impact on communication. A calm, uncluttered space can reduce sensory overload and improve focus. Minimize distractions like loud noises or bright lights. Speak in a soft, clear voice, ensuring your words are easy to understand. A quiet, comfortable space helps foster more effective and less stressful conversations. Reducing extraneous stimuli allows them to focus on the interaction itself. This simple change can make a world of difference.

Validation is crucial, even when the individual's statements are factually incorrect. Don't correct them aggressively; instead, acknowledge their feelings and perceptions. For example, if someone insists it's daytime when it's clearly night, respond with, "I understand you feel it's daytime. It's actually nighttime now, but we can look forward to the sun rising soon." This validation approach helps alleviate anxiety and avoid conflict, promoting a more positive interaction. It's not about deception; it's about emotional comfort.

Engage with local support groups. They offer invaluable practical advice, emotional support, and the chance to share experiences with others facing similar challenges. These groups offer a safe space to connect, learn from others, and reduce the burden of isolation. Don't underestimate the value of connecting with people who genuinely understand your situation. There's power in shared experience.

Remember that the person with Alzheimer's is still the same person they've always been, even though their cognitive abilities may have declined. Treat them with the same respect, dignity, and love you always have. Maintain eye contact, listen attentively, and demonstrate genuine interest in what they're trying to convey. Your empathy and compassion will reinforce the strength of your bond, enriching both your lives. Approaching each interaction with this perspective creates a foundation of mutual respect and understanding.

It's a journey, not a destination. There will be good days and bad days. Embrace the moments of connection, cherish the memories, and never underestimate the power of your love and support. Accept the challenges, and learn from each experience. Remember, you're not alone.

Professional assistance, support groups, and personal resilience are all vital components in navigating this challenging but ultimately rewarding path. There's hope, and your unwavering care makes a tangible difference. By fostering open communication and building strong relationships, you can improve the quality of life for both yourself and the individual living with Alzheimer's. This journey demands patience, understanding, and above all, love.

4.1 Effective Communication Tips

Effective communication is paramount in caring for someone with Alzheimer's. It's not just about conveying information; it's about building a connection, fostering understanding, and maintaining a sense of dignity. Remember, the person with Alzheimer's is still the same individual, albeit experiencing significant cognitive changes. Your approach should reflect that understanding, adapting to their evolving needs.

Patience is your most valuable tool. Avoid rushing the conversation or correcting them constantly. Instead, focus on their emotional state and respond accordingly. Sometimes, simply acknowledging their feelings, even if their recollection is inaccurate, is more effective than trying to force reality. A gentle touch, a reassuring smile, can speak volumes.

Use simple, clear language. Avoid jargon, complex sentences, or abstract concepts. Speak slowly and distinctly, using short, declarative sentences. Break down complex tasks or instructions into smaller, more manageable steps. For example, instead of saying, "Let's go for a walk in the park after lunch," try, "First, we'll eat lunch. Then, we'll put on our coats. After that, we'll go for a walk."

Engage their senses. Play familiar music, show family photographs, or use aromatherapy to trigger positive memories and reduce agitation. These sensory cues can be powerful communication aids, bridging the gap when words fail. Remember a familiar scent from their past, perhaps lavender or pipe tobacco. The smell itself might unlock positive memories and encourage communication.

Nonverbal cues are incredibly significant. Maintain eye contact, but don't stare intensely. Use a calm and reassuring tone of voice. Your body language should communicate patience, empathy, and respect. Approach them from the front, rather than startling them from behind. These simple actions can greatly reduce anxiety and promote a sense of security.

Focus on the present. Don't dwell on the past or try to correct their misrememberings. Instead, direct the conversation towards current activities or experiences. Discuss the weather, the food they're eating, or something they're currently enjoying. The present moment becomes the most important and relevant reality. Asking "What does this food taste like?" is preferable to discussing yesterday's events if they are confused.

Validate their feelings, even if their statements don't align with reality. Saying things like, "I understand you're feeling frustrated," or "That sounds upsetting," acknowledges their emotional experience without directly contradicting them. Focusing on the underlying emotional message— rather than the factual accuracy of their words — builds trust and rapport. This approach reduces tension and promotes a more peaceful interaction.

Choose the right time to communicate. Avoid overwhelming them with conversations during times of stress or fatigue. Pick a time when they are relatively relaxed and receptive. Consider the individual's daily routine and choose a time when they are most alert and engaged. Remember that overstimulation is a major factor in causing confusion.

Remember to take care of yourself. Caring for someone with Alzheimer's is emotionally and physically demanding. Make sure you have your support system in place, whether it's family, friends, or professional caregivers. Take breaks when needed, and don't hesitate to seek guidance from support groups or healthcare professionals. Your well-being is critical to your ability to provide effective care. Regular self-care can prevent caregiver burnout.

Learn about the disease. The more you understand Alzheimer's, the better equipped you are to handle challenges in communication. Attend workshops or consult specialists to gain a more thorough understanding of cognitive decline's impact on communication. Continuously updating your knowledge ensures you're using the most effective strategies. Recognising the progressive nature of the illness is crucial, allowing for timely adjustments to your communication approach. Professional resources can offer further training and support.

4.2 Building Positive Relationships

Strong, positive relationships are vital, not just for emotional well-being, but also for effective caregiving in Alzheimer's. Maintaining these connections provides a crucial source of comfort and support for both the person with Alzheimer's and their caregivers, easing the burden of this challenging journey. A supportive network can significantly enhance the quality of life for everyone involved.

Focusing on shared activities and memories is key. Think about the things the person enjoyed before the diagnosis – perhaps a specific type of music, a favorite hobby, or even a particular place they liked to visit. Reliving those moments, even in a simplified way, can stimulate positive emotions and strengthen your bond. Don't underestimate the power of a familiar song or a shared photograph in sparking recognition and joy. The goal isn't to fix what's lost; it's to celebrate what remains.

Patience, unwavering patience, is paramount. Communication changes as Alzheimer's progresses. Frustration is natural, but it's crucial to approach interactions with empathy and understanding. Remember, the person isn't intentionally being difficult; their brain is simply working differently. Responding with calmness and reassurance can defuse tense situations and create a more positive experience for both of you. Deep breaths, a change of scenery, or simply a quiet moment together can make a world of difference.

Nonverbal communication also plays a significant role. A gentle touch, a warm smile, or a comforting presence can convey care and understanding even when words fail. Physical affection can be immensely soothing, offering a connection beyond the limitations of verbal communication. These actions speak volumes, especially when words become difficult to comprehend or express. Observe their body language; it often speaks volumes about their comfort level and needs.

Maintaining a sense of normalcy is essential. Despite the challenges, try to integrate the person into everyday life as much as possible. Including them in activities, even simple ones, can foster a sense of purpose and belonging. It might be helping with simple chores, reading a book together, or listening to music. The key is to find activities tailored to their abilities and interests, ensuring participation is enjoyable and not overwhelming.

Seek out support from others. Caregiving for someone with Alzheimer's is demanding, and it's crucial to have a strong support system. Connect with other caregivers, either through support groups, online forums, or simply through trusted friends and family. Sharing experiences, offering mutual support, and receiving practical advice can make an immeasurable difference. Don't hesitate to ask for help; seeking support doesn't indicate weakness; it signifies strength and wisdom.

Remember to nurture your own well-being. Caregiver burnout is a serious concern. Prioritize self-care activities to prevent exhaustion and maintain your emotional and physical health. Engaging in activities you enjoy, maintaining healthy habits, and taking breaks when needed are crucial for your overall well-being and your capacity to provide effective care. Your well-being is inextricably linked to your ability to care for your loved one. Remember, you can't pour from an empty cup.

Professional assistance can be invaluable. Therapists specializing in Alzheimer's care and support groups provide invaluable resources and guidance, helping you navigate emotional challenges and learn effective coping strategies. Their expertise can equip you with tools and techniques to better manage stress, improve communication, and maintain a positive relationship. Don't hesitate to reach out for assistance. It's a sign of strength, not weakness.

Building positive relationships isn't merely about maintaining connections; it's about fostering a compassionate and supportive environment. This creates a sense of security and belonging, which are particularly crucial for someone living with Alzheimer's. Remember, the focus remains on cherishing the present, celebrating the personhood, and adapting to the ever-changing dynamics of the disease. The journey might be arduous, but the bonds you nurture will provide solace, strength, and a profound sense of purpose. It is a testament to the resilience of the human spirit and the enduring power of love. By prioritizing these relationships, you enrich the lives of both the person with Alzheimer's and yourself, transforming a challenging situation into one of meaningful connection and shared experience.

5 Maintaining Physical Health

Maintaining a healthy lifestyle is paramount, especially when caring for someone with Alzheimer's. Neglecting physical well-being can exacerbate symptoms and decrease overall quality of life for both the patient and the caregiver. Prioritizing nutrition, movement, and sleep are vital steps in managing the challenges of this disease.

A balanced diet rich in fruits, vegetables, whole grains, and lean protein provides essential nutrients for brain health. Focus on foods known to support cognitive function, such as blueberries, fatty fish, and nuts. Limit processed foods, sugary drinks, and saturated fats, as these can negatively impact overall health and potentially worsen cognitive decline. Regular meals, even if smaller and more frequent, can help maintain stable blood sugar levels, which is crucial for someone experiencing cognitive changes. Consult a registered dietitian or nutritionist to create a personalized meal plan that caters to the specific dietary needs and preferences of the individual with Alzheimer's. Remember, even small adjustments can make a difference. For example, offering visually appealing meals can stimulate appetite and improve food intake. Additionally, consider the textures of food, adapting it to match the patient's changing ability to chew and swallow. This may involve pureeing foods or opting for softer alternatives.

Regular physical activity is equally important. It doesn't need to be strenuous; gentle exercises like walking, chair exercises, or even simple range-of-motion movements can significantly improve circulation, mood, and sleep quality. Exercise reduces stress, a major factor contributing to caregiver burnout and the progression of Alzheimer's symptoms in the patient. Remember to consult a physician before starting any new exercise program, particularly for someone with Alzheimer's. They can help develop a safe and effective plan tailored to the individual's physical abilities and limitations. Consider incorporating activities the individual enjoys. A simple walk in a park or a light dance session can be far more beneficial than a forced routine. Adaptability and a focus on enjoyment are key. The emphasis should be on participation, not performance.

Establishing consistent sleep patterns is crucial. Sleep deprivation can exacerbate cognitive decline and increase agitation. Creating a relaxing bedtime routine can help induce sleep. This could include a warm bath, reading a familiar story, or listening to calming music. A comfortable and dark sleep environment is also essential. Avoid caffeine and alcohol close to bedtime. Maintain a regular sleep schedule, even on weekends, to regulate the body's natural sleep-wake cycle. If sleep disturbances persist, consult a physician or sleep specialist to rule out any underlying medical conditions and consider strategies such as cognitive behavioral therapy for insomnia.

Maintaining physical health in the context of Alzheimer's is not about achieving peak physical fitness but rather about supporting overall well-being. It's about providing a safe and stimulating environment that encourages gentle activity, supports nutritional needs, and promotes restful sleep. Each small step contributes to a better quality of life, not only for the individual with Alzheimer's but also for the caregivers navigating this journey. It's a continuous process of adaptation and adjustment, a collaborative effort requiring patience, understanding and the ongoing support of healthcare professionals. Remember that consistency and gentle encouragement are far more impactful than intense pressure or unrealistic goals. Focus on the progress, no matter how small, and celebrate the victories along the way. This approach fosters a positive and supportive environment, making the journey a little less challenging for everyone involved.

5.1 Nutrition & Diet

Maintaining a healthy diet is crucial for anyone, but it takes on added significance for individuals with Alzheimer's disease and their caregivers. Proper nutrition can't halt the disease's progression, but it can significantly impact the quality of life. Focusing on a balanced diet rich in specific nutrients is key to supporting cognitive function and overall well-being. We're not talking about restrictive diets here; rather, we're emphasizing the importance of incorporating certain foods into existing meal plans.

A diet rich in antioxidants, found in abundance in brightly colored fruits and vegetables like blueberries, strawberries, spinach, and kale, combats oxidative stress, a process believed to contribute to the development of Alzheimer's. These foods are packed with vitamins and minerals essential for brain health. Think of them as microscopic warriors, fighting off damaging free radicals within your brain cells. Regular consumption of these powerhouses can help protect against cellular damage.

Omega-3 fatty acids, primarily found in fatty fish such as salmon, tuna, and mackerel, are also vital. These essential fats are crucial for brain function and reduce inflammation, another factor linked to Alzheimer's progression. If you're not a fan of fish, consider incorporating flaxseeds or chia seeds into your diet—they're excellent vegetarian alternatives. Remember to consult a doctor or registered dietitian before making significant dietary changes, especially if you are already managing other health conditions. They can help tailor a nutritional plan that is appropriate for your individual needs and preferences.

Beyond specific nutrients, the overall structure of your diet matters. Prioritize whole, unprocessed foods, minimizing refined sugars, processed meats, and saturated and trans fats. These contribute to inflammation and can negatively impact overall health, potentially accelerating cognitive decline. Instead, load up on lean proteins, complex carbohydrates, and healthy fats. Think chicken breast, brown rice, and avocados – foods that provide sustained energy without the unhealthy sugar rush and crash. A balanced approach, focusing on nutrient density rather than caloric restriction, is crucial.

Hydration is often overlooked, yet it's vital for optimal brain function. Dehydration can lead to confusion and cognitive impairment, exacerbating symptoms. Aim to drink plenty of water throughout the day; consider carrying a water bottle and sipping on it regularly. It's a simple yet powerful step you can take to support your brain health. Incorporating foods with high water content, such as watermelon or cucumbers, can also contribute to your overall hydration. Listen to your body; thirst is a clear signal to drink.

Maintaining a consistent meal schedule is equally important, especially for individuals with Alzheimer's. Regular eating times help regulate blood sugar levels, preventing energy crashes that can lead to irritability and confusion. Structure and predictability are beneficial for those with cognitive impairments. Forgetting to eat is a common issue; setting reminders or establishing a routine with a caregiver can be invaluable. This structured approach provides both physical and mental benefits.

Social dining is another often-underestimated aspect. Sharing meals with loved ones fosters connection and reduces feelings of isolation, which can positively impact mood and cognitive function. Mealtimes shouldn't just be about nourishment; they should also be opportunities for social interaction and emotional support. Remember, a positive and supportive environment is an integral part of Alzheimer's care.

Lastly, it's crucial to be patient and understanding. Dietary changes take time to implement and adjust, especially for individuals with Alzheimer's. Expect setbacks and be prepared to adapt your approach as needed. It's a journey, not a race. Celebrate small victories and continue to find ways to incorporate healthy eating habits into daily routines. Remember that consistency is key; even small, consistent efforts can make a significant difference over time. Involve your loved ones, making meal preparation and eating a collaborative process. Working together promotes a sense of shared responsibility and encourages adherence to healthier eating patterns. With patience, persistence, and a supportive environment, it's possible to make sustainable changes that positively impact overall well-being and potentially slow cognitive decline.

5.2 Exercise & Activity

Regular physical activity is crucial for individuals with Alzheimer's, offering benefits that extend beyond simple fitness. Maintaining mobility and preventing muscle atrophy are key, significantly impacting their independence and overall quality of life. Even simple movements can have a surprisingly positive effect, fostering a sense of accomplishment and combating the feelings of helplessness that can accompany the disease. These small victories, however modest, contribute to a more positive self-image.

Structured exercise programs, tailored to the individual's abilities, are highly beneficial. These programs should include a combination of aerobic exercises like gentle walking or swimming, strength training exercises utilizing light weights or resistance bands, and flexibility exercises such as stretching and yoga. Remember to consult a physician before starting any new exercise regimen, especially for individuals with existing health conditions, and always prioritize safety.

Consider the environment when planning activities. A safe, familiar space minimizes anxiety and encourages participation. Music can also enhance the experience, providing a calming or motivating influence depending on the chosen selection. Even something as simple as a walk in a garden, providing visual stimulation and a change of scenery, can be incredibly therapeutic and engaging.

Beyond formal exercise programs, encourage daily activities that promote movement. Simple tasks such as gardening, light housework, or even dancing can significantly contribute to overall physical activity. These tasks can be adapted to suit varying levels of ability and cognitive function. Maintaining engagement is key, keeping them active and preventing further decline. Furthermore, these activities can foster a sense of purpose and contribution, improving their self-esteem.

Social interaction is an often overlooked component of physical health. Group activities, such as chair yoga or walking groups, offer both physical and social benefits. The social interaction combats isolation, a common problem among those living with Alzheimer's, and boosts their mood. Shared experiences and interaction help maintain cognitive function and offer a vital sense of community. The support they receive from others involved significantly aids their journey.

Remember, the goal isn't to achieve peak physical fitness. The focus should be on maintaining mobility, strength, and flexibility, while encouraging social interaction and engagement. Regular monitoring of progress is essential to adapt the exercise program as the disease progresses. This adaptive approach ensures the individual continues to benefit from the activities and avoids frustration caused by inappropriate challenges. Flexibility is paramount.

Observe your loved one closely for signs of fatigue or discomfort during activities. Adjust the intensity and duration of activities as needed, always prioritizing their comfort and safety. Patience and understanding are essential throughout the process, celebrating every achievement, no matter how small. Positive reinforcement encourages continued participation and fosters a sense of accomplishment, combating feelings of inadequacy and frustration. Celebrating progress, however minimal, is critical.

The benefits of physical activity for individuals with Alzheimer's extend beyond physical health. It helps maintain cognitive function, improves sleep quality, and reduces anxiety and depression. Furthermore, regular exercise can have a significant impact on mood, promoting overall well-being. The combined effect of physical and mental stimulation is essential for enhancing their quality of life.

It's crucial to remember that consistency is key. Regular, even if short, periods of activity are far more beneficial than sporadic bursts of intense exercise. Start slowly, gradually increasing the intensity and duration of activities as tolerated. This gradual approach prevents overwhelming the individual and ensures they remain engaged and motivated. Consistency builds a routine which is calming and supportive to their condition.

Finally, incorporate these activities into the individual's daily routine. This makes participation easier and less disruptive to their established patterns. Making exercise a natural part of their day ensures it's less of a chore and more of an enjoyable experience. Remember, a positive attitude significantly influences their success and enjoyment of the activities and this positive reinforcement is key to ongoing success. Remember, even small improvements can have significant long-term benefits.

5.3 Sleep Hygiene

Sufficient, restorative sleep is paramount for individuals with Alzheimer's, impacting cognitive function, mood regulation, and overall health. Sleep disturbances are common in Alzheimer's, manifesting as insomnia, sleep apnea, or disrupted sleep cycles. These disruptions can exacerbate cognitive decline and behavioral issues, creating a significant challenge for both the patient and their caregivers. Addressing sleep problems effectively requires a multi-pronged approach focusing on environmental modifications, behavioral strategies, and, when necessary, medical intervention.

Creating a conducive sleep environment is the first crucial step. This involves optimizing the bedroom for sleep. Ensure the room is dark, quiet, and cool. Consider using blackout curtains, earplugs, or a white noise machine to minimize external distractions. A comfortable, supportive mattress and bedding are essential. The bedroom should be solely associated with sleep and relaxation; avoid using it for work or other stimulating activities. Regularly airing the room and maintaining a consistent temperature can also contribute to improved sleep quality.

The consistent routine of these changes over time will create a better sleeping environment.

Establishing a regular sleep schedule is equally important. Try to maintain a consistent wake-up and bedtime, even on weekends, to regulate the body's natural sleep-wake cycle. Regularity helps synchronize the circadian rhythm, promoting better sleep onset and maintaining a more consistent sleep pattern throughout the night. Avoid napping during the day, particularly later in the afternoon or evening, as this can interfere with nighttime sleep. This structured approach is particularly beneficial for those with Alzheimer's, whose sleep patterns may already be disrupted. The consistency of the schedule is key to the body's ability to adjust and find a normal sleep cycle.

Before bedtime, engage in relaxing activities that signal to the body it is time to wind down. This could include a warm bath, reading a book, listening to calming music, or gentle stretching. Avoid strenuous exercise, stimulating conversations, or screen time close to bedtime as these can interfere with sleep onset. These activities help promote relaxation and reduce the stimulating activity of the mind, which is vital before sleep. Avoid caffeinated or alcoholic beverages several hours before bedtime, as these substances can disrupt sleep patterns and negatively impact sleep quality. Creating a personalized relaxation routine is essential to calm the mind and body for sleep.

Dietary considerations also play a significant role in sleep quality. A healthy, balanced diet contributes to overall well-being and can positively influence sleep. Regular mealtimes and avoiding heavy meals or large amounts of fluids before bed can minimize nighttime awakenings caused by indigestion or bathroom trips. The correct amount of fluids and food eaten during the day are very important, as a late dinner is a common sleep problem for individuals of all ages. Ensuring a balanced diet throughout the day can lead to better quality sleep.

If sleep problems persist despite implementing these strategies, consult a physician or sleep specialist. Underlying medical conditions such as sleep apnea, restless legs syndrome, or other neurological issues may be contributing to sleep disturbances. A thorough medical evaluation can help identify these conditions and recommend appropriate treatment options. These conditions can be easily treated with medical intervention. They can be caused by several reasons, from medical conditions to mental illnesses. A diagnosis will allow proper treatment.

Medication should only be considered as a last resort, after attempting non-pharmacological approaches. While some medications can improve sleep, they also carry the risk of side effects, especially for individuals with Alzheimer's who are often on multiple medications. Always consult a physician before introducing any new medications, carefully weighing the potential benefits against the risks. The use of medication to treat sleep problems in Alzheimer's disease should always be carefully monitored and adjusted as needed. The treatment should always consider any possible side effects the medication may have on the patient.

Beyond managing sleep disturbances, promoting daytime activity and physical exercise is crucial. Regular physical activity helps regulate sleep-wake cycles, reducing daytime sleepiness and promoting better sleep at night. Activities should be tailored to the individual's abilities and preferences, focusing on safety and enjoyment. Simple activities, such as walking, gentle stretching, or chair exercises, can be beneficial. The appropriate amount of exercise varies from person to person and must be monitored and adjusted to avoid any risks of injuries. Appropriate exercise improves sleep quality and reduces daytime sleepiness. Caregivers play a critical role in supporting individuals with Alzheimer's to establish and maintain good sleep hygiene. They can provide support in implementing the strategies discussed above, creating a supportive and consistent sleep environment, and advocating for professional medical assistance when needed. Patience, understanding, and consistent support are essential in helping their loved ones achieve better sleep and improved quality of life. A balanced approach considering environmental, behavioral, and medical interventions is essential for managing sleep problems successfully. The caregiver's support is invaluable and crucial for effective management.

6 Advanced Stages & End-of-Life Care

Managing symptoms becomes paramount in advanced Alzheimer's. Pain, agitation, and difficulty swallowing are common, requiring careful monitoring and tailored interventions. Non-pharmacological approaches, like soothing music, aromatherapy, and gentle touch, can sometimes alleviate distress. Pharmacological interventions, however, may be necessary to manage more severe symptoms. Antipsychotics, for example, might be used cautiously to address agitation, but their use should be carefully weighed against potential side effects, such as increased risk of falls and stroke. Regular reassessment of medication effectiveness and side effects is crucial. Pain management involves identifying the source of pain—whether it's related to arthritis, pressure sores, or other conditions—and then choosing the most appropriate treatment, ranging from over-the-counter analgesics to stronger prescription medications, always under the guidance of a physician. A multidisciplinary approach involving doctors, nurses, and therapists is essential for optimal symptom control and compassionate care. The goal is not to cure the disease, but to maximize comfort and quality of life during this challenging phase.

The transition into the later stages often necessitates a shift in care settings. Home care might become increasingly challenging as the person's needs intensify. Respite care, providing temporary relief for caregivers, can be invaluable in preventing burnout and maintaining the caregiver's own well-being. Assisted living facilities offer a structured environment with more support for daily tasks, while nursing homes provide comprehensive 24-hour care for individuals with complex needs. These transitions aren't easy; they require careful planning and consideration of the individual's preferences and the family's capabilities. Open communication with healthcare professionals is key to making informed decisions about the best placement options. A thorough assessment of the individual's needs, both physical and cognitive, guides the selection of an appropriate care setting, ensuring a safe and supportive environment. The goal is always to maintain dignity and provide the best possible quality of life, adapting the care setting as the individual's needs change.

Hospice care plays a crucial role in the end-of-life phase of Alzheimer's. It focuses on providing comfort and support, rather than curative treatment. Hospice services can be delivered in various settings, including the patient's home, nursing homes, or dedicated hospice facilities. They often involve a team of professionals, including doctors, nurses, social workers, and chaplains, who work collaboratively to address the physical, emotional, and spiritual needs of the patient and their family. Palliative care shares many similarities with hospice care, focusing on relieving suffering and improving quality of life. However, palliative care can be provided at any stage of the illness, unlike hospice care, which is typically initiated when a prognosis of six months or less remains. Both palliative and hospice care emphasize a holistic approach to care, prioritizing the individual's comfort and dignity in their final days. Access to these services is essential for providing compassionate and respectful end-of-life care, helping both the patient and their loved ones navigate this difficult period with grace and support.

One of the most significant aspects of end-of-life care involves addressing the emotional and spiritual needs of both the patient and their family. This often requires sensitive communication and a compassionate approach. For patients, maintaining a sense of comfort and familiarity can help ease anxiety and distress. Listening to their favorite music, sharing cherished memories, or engaging in quiet activities that they once enjoyed can create a sense of peace. For families, providing emotional support, offering practical assistance, and helping them navigate the grieving process are essential components of compassionate care. Grief counseling, support groups, and bereavement services can offer invaluable assistance during this challenging time. Respecting the individual's wishes and preferences, even in their inability to express them explicitly, is paramount. A careful consideration of advance directives, such as living wills and durable power of attorney, helps ensure that the patient's end-of-life wishes are honored, promoting peace of mind for both the patient and their loved ones. It's a testament to the value of human connection and the profound impact of empathy and understanding. Open communication between the family and the care team is indispensable for coordinating care and providing optimal support throughout this journey.

Preparing for the end-of-life phase often involves complex legal and financial considerations. Advance care planning, which includes creating legal documents like living wills and durable powers of attorney, is crucial for ensuring that the patient's wishes are respected concerning their medical care and financial matters. These documents allow individuals to designate a trusted person to make decisions on their behalf if they become incapacitated. Discussions about funeral arrangements and estate planning are also important. Open and honest conversations with family members about these issues can alleviate stress and ensure that arrangements are made according to the patient's wishes. Healthcare professionals can provide valuable guidance on these matters, helping families navigate the legal and financial aspects of end-of-life care. Financial planning, including reviewing insurance policies and exploring options for long-term care coverage, is also vital in ensuring financial security for both the patient and their family during this challenging period. Understanding the options available and planning proactively can significantly reduce stress and improve the overall quality of end-of-life care.

6.1 Symptom Management

Managing symptoms in the advanced stages of Alzheimer's requires a multifaceted approach focusing on comfort and quality of life. Pain management, for instance, is crucial. Often, individuals experience discomfort from conditions like arthritis or other age-related ailments, and these pains can be exacerbated by the disease itself, leading to increased agitation and distress. Regular assessment of pain levels, using validated pain scales tailored for individuals with cognitive impairment, is essential, followed by the appropriate pharmacological or non-pharmacological interventions like heat packs or massage therapy under medical supervision. Never underestimate the power of simple comfort measures. A warm bath, soothing music, or a gentle touch can significantly alleviate discomfort and anxiety.

Dealing with behavioral issues poses another major challenge. Wandering, aggression, or agitation are common symptoms that can significantly impact both the individual's well-being and the caregiver's ability to provide care. It's vital to identify triggers for these behaviors – perhaps hunger, thirst, discomfort, or unmet needs. Environmental modifications, such as reducing clutter or increasing lighting, can sometimes help reduce agitation. Strategies like validating the individual's feelings, even if their statements don't seem entirely logical, can also be effective in calming them. Medication may be necessary in some cases, but should always be considered a last resort and implemented under the guidance of a medical professional. Remember that each individual's needs are unique, and what works for one person may not work for another. The goal is finding the most appropriate and compassionate strategies for managing these challenges, thereby preserving the person's dignity.

Sleep disturbances are prevalent in Alzheimer's disease, disrupting both the patient's and the caregiver's routines. Insomnia, daytime sleepiness, and frequent nighttime awakenings are common, impacting mood, cognition, and overall health. Establishing a regular sleep-wake cycle, creating a calming bedtime routine, and ensuring a comfortable sleep environment are crucial. Avoiding caffeine and alcohol before bedtime and providing ample opportunities for daytime activity can improve sleep quality. However, if these measures are insufficient, a healthcare professional should be consulted to rule out other medical conditions and consider appropriate medication, always mindful of potential side effects. Prioritize creating a safe and peaceful environment conducive to restful sleep; it's a cornerstone of managing the overall quality of life during this challenging phase.

Appetite changes and nutritional deficits are also common. Difficulty swallowing, reduced taste perception, or forgetfulness about eating can lead to malnutrition and dehydration. Frequent small meals, easily digestible foods, and assistance with eating may be needed. Nutritional supplements can be beneficial under medical supervision to address any nutritional deficiencies. Hydration is crucial, offering regular sips of fluids throughout the day. Make mealtimes as enjoyable and comfortable as possible, utilizing sensory stimulation where appropriate, such as appealing aromas and textures, and avoiding distractions. Regular monitoring of weight and nutritional intake is necessary to prevent serious health complications associated with poor nutrition. Remember to consult a dietitian to develop a tailored nutritional plan.

Continence issues, including urinary and bowel incontinence, can significantly affect the dignity and well-being of individuals with Alzheimer's, adding another layer of complexity to caregiving. Maintaining good hygiene practices, regular toileting schedules, and using absorbent products can help manage incontinence. Consulting a healthcare professional to rule out other medical causes and evaluate potential medication options is essential. Effective communication with the individual, understanding their nonverbal cues, and providing positive reinforcement can also ease the emotional impact of these challenges. Above all, maintain a respectful and sensitive approach, recognizing the patient's vulnerability and preserving their dignity throughout this difficult period. The goal is to provide comfort and maintain the highest level of personal dignity as possible in every aspect of care.

Managing these symptoms requires patience, empathy, and a collaborative effort between caregivers, healthcare professionals, and family members. Regular communication with the healthcare team is essential to monitor the effectiveness of interventions and adjust the care plan as needed. Remember, the goal isn't to cure the disease but to improve the person's quality of life, minimize suffering, and provide comfort and support during the final stages of Alzheimer's. This holistic approach, combining medical interventions with compassionate care, is fundamental to ensuring the best possible outcome for both the individual with Alzheimer's and their loved ones. Never hesitate to seek guidance and support from professionals and support groups; you are not alone in this journey.

6.2 Hospice & Palliative Care

The transition to hospice care for an Alzheimer's patient is often a difficult decision, but one that can profoundly impact the quality of life for both the patient and their family. It signifies a shift in focus, from attempting to cure or significantly delay the disease's progression, to prioritizing comfort, pain management, and emotional support. This is not about giving up; it's about embracing a new phase where the emphasis is on dignity and peace.

Hospice care isn't just a place; it's a philosophy. It's a holistic approach that addresses the physical, emotional, and spiritual needs of the patient, as well as the needs of their loved ones. A dedicated team, including nurses, doctors, social workers, chaplains, and volunteers, works collaboratively to create a personalized care plan tailored to the individual's unique requirements. This comprehensive approach considers the patient's preferences and ensures they receive compassionate care in their preferred setting, whether it's at home, in a hospice facility, or in a nursing home.

Effective pain management is paramount in hospice care for Alzheimer's patients. Since many individuals with advanced-stage Alzheimer's can't verbally communicate their pain, skilled professionals utilize observation and assessment tools to identify discomfort. This often involves monitoring subtle changes in behavior, such as restlessness, agitation, or changes in appetite or sleep patterns. Medication is adjusted accordingly to ensure the patient's comfort and to manage other challenging symptoms like agitation, anxiety, or depression. The goal is to minimize suffering, allowing the patient to experience their remaining time with as much peace and tranquility as possible.

Beyond pain management, a crucial aspect of hospice care is addressing the emotional and spiritual well-being of both the patient and the family. This might involve providing emotional support, facilitating family meetings to discuss end-of-life decisions and wishes, offering spiritual guidance if desired, or simply providing a listening ear. Hospice workers understand the profound emotional toll that caring for someone with a debilitating illness can take, and they offer respite and support to ease the burden on caregivers. This emotional support is as vital as any medication, allowing families to cope with the emotional complexities of this journey, providing a safe space for grieving and healing to begin even before the patient's passing.

Palliative care, while sometimes used interchangeably with hospice care, has a slightly different focus. It encompasses a broader range of services, available at any stage of the illness, not just the final stages. Palliative care emphasizes symptom relief, improving quality of life, and supporting both the patient and their family. It can be provided concurrently with other medical treatments, aiming to enhance comfort and well-being throughout the disease progression. Think of it as a complement to curative treatments, improving the patient's overall experience, regardless of their prognosis. One might utilize palliative care strategies to manage challenging behaviors, improve communication, or provide respite care for overwhelmed caregivers long before hospice care becomes necessary. This proactive approach can greatly enhance the patient's quality of life and support the entire family unit.

Choosing hospice or palliative care is a personal decision. Families need to weigh several factors, including the patient's prognosis, their preferences, and the available resources. Open communication with the healthcare team is crucial, ensuring that everyone involved understands the patient's needs and goals. This collaborative approach ensures that the patient receives the best possible care, tailored to their unique circumstances and preferences, fostering a sense of dignity, peace, and comfort during a challenging time. The resources available through hospice and palliative care, both in terms of physical care and emotional support, make a profound difference in the final chapter of an individual's life, alleviating suffering and allowing for a more peaceful and meaningful transition.

Accessing hospice care often involves a referral from a physician, who will assess the patient's condition and determine if they meet the eligibility criteria. This usually involves a life expectancy of six months or less if the disease runs its natural course. However, it's vital to initiate conversations early, as this allows ample time for planning and preparation. Discussing preferences for end-of-life care, completing advance directives like living wills, and arranging for practical matters such as financial arrangements and legal documents are all crucial aspects of the process. These preparations provide a sense of control and help families navigate the complex emotional and logistical challenges of this phase.

Remember, seeking support is a sign of strength, not weakness. Utilizing the resources available through hospice and palliative care empowers families to provide the best possible care and support for their loved ones during their final journey. Don't hesitate to reach out to healthcare professionals, support groups, or other resources available in your community. It's vital to have a team of professionals and loved ones who understand the nuances of Alzheimer's and provide appropriate support through the final stages. The goal is to make the transition as peaceful and dignified as possible, both for the patient and for those who love them. This comprehensive approach to end-of-life care for Alzheimer's patients not only focuses on comfort and symptom management but also on preserving the dignity and celebrating the life of the individual.

7 Finding Hope & Acceptance

The journey with Alzheimer's is undeniably difficult, a relentless erosion of memory and familiarity. Yet, within this challenging landscape, hope and acceptance are not merely abstract concepts; they are vital tools for navigating this path, for both the person with Alzheimer's and their loved ones. Finding them requires a conscious effort, a willingness to embrace the present moment while acknowledging the past and the uncertainties of the future.

Acceptance, however, isn't about resignation; it's about recognizing the reality of the situation without allowing it to define your entire existence. It's about acknowledging the disease's impact without surrendering to despair. This acceptance allows for a shift in focus, from fighting against the inevitable to finding meaning and joy in the moments that remain. This might mean celebrating small victories – a shared laugh, a moment of recognition, or simply a peaceful afternoon together. These small moments, often overlooked in the midst of the challenges, become precious treasures when viewed through the lens of acceptance.

Emotional processing is crucial. Allowing yourself, and the person with Alzheimer's, to feel the full spectrum of emotions – sadness, anger, frustration, fear – is a necessary step. Suppressing these feelings only prolongs the suffering. Seeking professional support, whether through therapy, counseling, or support groups, can provide a safe and structured environment to process these complex emotions. Talking about your feelings, sharing your experiences, and hearing from others who understand can make a profound difference in your ability to cope. Remember, you are not alone in this journey.

Spiritual support can offer a powerful source of comfort and strength. For many, faith provides a framework for understanding suffering, finding meaning in the face of adversity, and fostering a sense of peace. Whether through prayer, meditation, or connecting with a religious community, spiritual practices can offer solace and guidance during challenging times. This does not necessitate a specific religious belief; it's about finding a sense of connection to something larger than oneself, a source of strength and hope that transcends the immediate reality of the disease.

Celebrating life and memories is an essential act of remembrance and affirmation. Sharing photographs, reminiscing about shared experiences, and creating new memories—however small—can help preserve a sense of connection and continuity. Consider creating a memory book filled with pictures and stories, or perhaps planning special outings that cater to the person's current abilities and interests. These activities aren't just about preserving the past; they are about creating meaningful moments in the present, moments that can provide comfort and joy for both the person with Alzheimer's and their loved ones.

Support groups provide an invaluable resource, offering a space for caregivers and families to connect with others who understand the unique challenges of Alzheimer's. Sharing experiences, offering mutual support, and learning from one another can alleviate feelings of isolation and provide practical advice. These groups offer a sense of community, a reminder that you are not alone in navigating this journey. The shared experiences and understanding offered by fellow caregivers can be incredibly powerful.

Looking ahead, even when faced with an uncertain future, is not about denying the present reality but about focusing on what you can control. This might involve making plans for the future, such as establishing legal documents, securing financial resources, or arranging for long-term care. However, looking ahead also means cultivating hope – hope for moments of connection, hope for moments of joy, hope for finding peace and acceptance in the face of a challenging situation. Hope isn't about denying the disease; it's about finding strength in the face of adversity, embracing the present, and finding meaning in every moment. Remembering that each day holds the potential for connection, for love, and for small moments of happiness is key to sustaining hope. This journey may be arduous, but it's also a journey that can be navigated with grace, with compassion, and with a steadfast focus on the importance of hope and acceptance.

7.1 Emotional Processing

The journey with Alzheimer's isn't just about medical facts; it's deeply emotional. For the person diagnosed, the experience can range from bewilderment and fear to profound sadness and anger, as their memories and sense of self gradually fade. Understanding these feelings, validating them, and creating space for their expression is paramount. Encourage open dialogue, even if responses are fragmented or seemingly illogical. Remember, the emotional experience is as real as the physical changes.

For caregivers, the emotional toll is immense. It's a relentless cycle of worry, frustration, and grief. They may experience a sense of loss even before the person with Alzheimer's is gone. Their own identity can become blurred under the weight of responsibility. Seeking professional support, connecting with support groups, or simply allowing oneself time for self-care is not a sign of weakness but a necessity for survival. Prioritizing mental health doesn't diminish the love and commitment shown to the patient; it strengthens it.

Recognizing the emotional landscape, both for the individual with Alzheimer's and their caregivers, requires patience and understanding. It's about acknowledging the full spectrum of emotions, allowing space for tears, laughter, anger, or even quiet moments of reflection. There is no single "right" way to feel. Avoid judgment, focus on empathy. Creating a supportive environment, one built on trust and acceptance, becomes crucial.

Don't underestimate the power of reminiscing. Sharing old photographs, listening to favourite music, or recounting cherished memories can be profoundly therapeutic. These activities tap into preserved cognitive functions, providing moments of connection and joy. They can soothe anxieties and provide a sense of continuity amidst the changes. Consider creating memory boxes filled with meaningful objects, or even compiling a personalized photo album.

Professional guidance can prove invaluable in navigating these emotional complexities. Therapists specializing in Alzheimer's care can provide specialized coping mechanisms and strategies for both patients and caregivers. They offer a safe space to express feelings and explore strategies for managing stress and grief. Moreover, they can help families understand the disease's emotional impact and learn how to best respond. Don't hesitate to seek professional help; it's a sign of strength, not weakness.

The emotional journey with Alzheimer's is unpredictable. There will be moments of intense sadness, moments of unexpected joy, moments of frustration, and moments of peaceful acceptance. Each moment holds value, each emotion is valid. The key lies in learning to navigate these emotional waves with empathy, understanding, and a steadfast commitment to compassion. This isn't just about managing a disease; it's about supporting a person, their memories, and their dignity throughout a challenging period. It's about fostering hope in the midst of uncertainty. Remember, it's okay to feel a full range of emotions; allowing yourself to process them authentically is part of the healing process. Seeking support and allowing yourself to grieve are important steps in accepting this journey and finding hope along the way. Connecting with others facing similar challenges can provide invaluable solace and strength. Remember, you're not alone.

7.2 Spiritual Support

Many find solace in their faith or spiritual beliefs during challenging times, and Alzheimer's is undoubtedly a challenging time. This journey, for both the person with Alzheimer's and their caregivers, can evoke a profound sense of loss and uncertainty, making spiritual exploration a vital coping mechanism. For some, this might involve strengthening their connection with an existing faith community, attending services, or engaging in prayer or meditation. Others might find comfort in exploring new spiritual paths or practices such as mindfulness or yoga, which can provide a sense of calm and centeredness amidst the chaos.

The importance of personalized spiritual support cannot be overstated. What resonates deeply with one individual may not resonate with another. There's no one-size-fits-all approach. A caregiver's role extends beyond the practical; it includes understanding and respecting the patient's spiritual needs, even if those needs change or evolve over time. Perhaps the patient once found comfort in long church services but now finds shorter, quieter moments of reflection more beneficial. The key is adaptability and empathy.

For caregivers themselves, the emotional toll of caring for someone with Alzheimer's can be immense. Burnout is a very real concern, and spiritual practices can act as a buffer against the emotional strain. Regular meditation, prayer, or time spent in nature can offer moments of peace and replenishment, enabling caregivers to face the challenges with renewed strength and resilience. Remember, it is perfectly acceptable—even necessary—for caregivers to seek their own spiritual guidance and support during this journey. This is not selfish; it is self-preservation, allowing them to continue providing the best possible care for their loved one.

Connecting with faith-based organizations or support groups specifically designed for caregivers of Alzheimer's patients can be incredibly valuable. These communities offer shared experiences, emotional support, and practical advice from individuals navigating similar situations. The sense of belonging and shared understanding can be profoundly healing, lessening the feeling of isolation that often accompanies caregiving. These organizations frequently offer resources such as grief counseling, spiritual guidance, and workshops on coping strategies.

Beyond organized religious institutions, the natural world can also offer a potent form of spiritual solace. Spending time in nature—whether a quiet walk in the park, a visit to a garden, or simply sitting under a tree—can be a deeply restorative experience. The tranquility of nature can help to calm the mind, reduce stress, and foster a sense of peace and connection. Encourage the individual with Alzheimer's to participate in these activities, as the sensory experiences can be beneficial, even in advanced stages of the disease. Simple activities like touching leaves or feeling the sun on their skin can be grounding and soothing.

The exploration of art, music, or creative expression can also serve as a powerful spiritual outlet. Music therapy, in particular, has been shown to have beneficial effects on individuals with Alzheimer's, often triggering positive memories and emotional responses. Engaging in art therapy can also be a valuable tool for self-expression and emotional processing, allowing both patients and caregivers to express feelings that may be difficult to articulate through words. The creation of art itself can be a meditative and therapeutic experience, regardless of artistic skill.

In the later stages of Alzheimer's, when communication becomes more challenging, non-verbal forms of spiritual expression become increasingly important. Gentle touch, a comforting presence, or simply sitting quietly with the individual can convey love, care, and spiritual connection. These acts of presence are often more powerful than words in offering solace and peace. Remember that spiritual support isn't solely about grand gestures or religious rituals; it's about fostering a sense of connection, meaning, and peace in whatever ways feel most comforting and appropriate for the individual.

Ultimately, spiritual support within the context of Alzheimer's is a deeply personal journey. There's no right or wrong way to approach it. The aim is to find what brings comfort, meaning, and solace to both the person with Alzheimer's and their caregivers. Open communication, empathy, and a willingness to explore different avenues of spiritual expression are crucial for navigating this sensitive and challenging aspect of the disease. Remember to be patient, understanding, and adaptable as needs change throughout the progression of the disease. The journey may be challenging, but by fostering spiritual well-being, you can enhance quality of life and find strength amidst the difficulties.

7.3 Celebrating Life & Memories

Focusing on the positive aspects of a person's life, even in the face of Alzheimer's, is crucial. It's not about ignoring the disease; it's about enriching the present and honoring the past. Creating a vibrant tapestry of cherished memories can bring comfort and joy, providing a powerful counterpoint to the challenges of the illness. Remember, those memories are not just for the person with Alzheimer's; they're vital for the caregivers too, offering a lifeline to connection and shared history.

Photographs are invaluable. Gather family photos, old yearbooks, vacation snapshots – anything that evokes happy times. Arrange these photos chronologically, creating a visual timeline of their life. As you go through them together, narrate the stories behind each image, recalling details and anecdotes. Even if the person with Alzheimer's doesn't fully grasp every detail, the familiar faces and settings can stimulate recognition and emotional responses, fostering a sense of connection and belonging. If they are able, invite them to contribute to the story, prompting memories with gentle questions.

Music holds a special place in memory. Familiar songs often remain accessible long after other cognitive abilities have declined. Create personalized playlists of their favorite music from different periods of their life. Play these songs regularly, observing their reactions. Music can unlock memories and emotions, bringing a sense of peace and familiarity to their day. Perhaps you might sing along together, sharing the joy of music as a shared experience that transcends words. Consider creating a memory box containing meaningful objects that evoke particular memories. These could include old letters, awards, photographs, or even items from hobbies and pastimes.

Consider creating a life story book. This is a wonderful way to preserve memories and celebrate a life well-lived. You can include photos, stories, and anecdotes from different stages of their life, highlighting personal achievements, relationships, and cherished moments. This book becomes a tangible representation of their life journey, providing a source of comfort and reflection for both the person with Alzheimer's and their loved ones. Even small details—a favorite food, a cherished vacation spot, a beloved pet—can evoke powerful emotions and rekindle precious memories. The process of creating this book can be just as valuable as the final product, becoming a shared experience of reminiscing and bonding.

Engage in activities they enjoyed before the diagnosis. These might include simple tasks like gardening, knitting, or listening to audiobooks, or more involved activities such as playing board games or watching old movies. Adapting activities to their current capabilities is crucial, always focusing on participation and enjoyment rather than perfect performance. The goal is to facilitate engagement, to keep their minds and spirits stimulated. The sense of accomplishment, however small, can be incredibly rewarding. If mobility is an issue, consider adapting activities to a seated position.

Remember, celebrating life and memories isn't just about looking back; it's also about creating new ones. While cognitive abilities may diminish, the capacity for emotional connection and enjoyment often remains. Focus on shared experiences in the present moment: reading together, enjoying a meal, listening to music, or simply holding hands. These simple acts of connection can be profoundly meaningful, creating new memories that contribute to a richer, more fulfilling life. These shared moments are valuable treasures, even if only one party consciously remembers them in the future.

Consider involving other family members and friends in this process. Shared memories can strengthen bonds and provide a sense of community and support. Organize family gatherings where stories are shared and photos are viewed. Invite others to contribute to the life story book or to share their cherished memories of the individual. This collaborative effort can be incredibly enriching, creating a shared legacy of love and remembrance. A shared experience of reminiscing is a valuable bonding experience, fostering connection and understanding. Encouraging participation in creating a memory tapestry is an important step in providing comfort and continuity for all involved. The collective effort underscores the power of connection and shared history in navigating the challenges of Alzheimer's disease. Each contribution adds a layer to a vibrant narrative of their life.

7.4 Support Groups

Support groups offer a lifeline, a haven where the shared experience of Alzheimer's disease transforms isolation into connection. They aren't just about sharing stories; they are about finding strength in numbers, learning from others' triumphs and struggles, and discovering that you're not alone in navigating this challenging journey.

For caregivers, the emotional toll of Alzheimer's is immense. The constant demands, the witnessing of a loved one's decline, the sheer exhaustion—these factors can lead to burnout, depression, and feelings of helplessness. Support groups offer a safe space to express these emotions, to share frustrations without judgment, and to find solace in knowing that others understand. It's a chance to vent, to cry, to simply be heard, and in that shared vulnerability, strength is discovered. Practical advice is exchanged – tips on managing challenging behaviors, strategies for communication, resources for respite care – turning a space of shared hardship into a springboard for improved coping skills.

Patients, too, benefit immensely from support groups. While their cognitive abilities may fluctuate, the sense of community, the feeling of being understood, the simple act of being present with others facing similar challenges can profoundly impact their quality of life. These groups may not always offer tangible solutions to memory loss, but they provide a crucial sense of belonging, an affirmation that their experience is valid, and a space where memories and moments of joy can still be celebrated. It's a reminder that despite the disease, their identity and worth remain intact. Sometimes, simple activities within the group, like reminiscing over old photographs or sharing favorite songs, become potent tools for preserving a sense of self and connection with the past.

Finding the right support group is crucial. Some are specifically designed for caregivers, others for patients, and still others cater to both. Some focus on specific aspects of care, such as managing challenging behaviors or communicating effectively, while others provide a more general forum for sharing experiences and emotional support. It is essential to research groups in your area, considering the specific needs and preferences of yourself or your loved one. Online support groups offer a valuable alternative, especially for individuals with limited mobility or those living in geographically isolated areas. These virtual communities provide similar benefits – the comfort of shared experiences, the exchange of practical advice, and the sense of belonging – without the logistical constraints of in-person meetings.

However, finding the right fit is vital; a group that feels judgmental or lacks empathy will not be beneficial. It's essential to find a group that aligns with your personal values, provides a supportive environment, and offers practical and emotional support. If the first group you try doesn't quite work, keep searching; the right support group can become an invaluable resource, a source of strength and resilience during the difficult journey of Alzheimer's. It becomes a crucial companion, a journey shared with individuals who understand the unique struggles, joys, and profound impact of this illness. The shared experience transforms what might feel like isolation into a space of collective strength and understanding.

Remember, participation in a support group isn't a sign of weakness; it's a proactive step towards self-care, emotional well-being, and gaining valuable insight and support. It's a recognition of the immense challenges associated with Alzheimer's and a commitment to seeking the help you need and deserve. The strength derived from these connections is immeasurable, providing a much-needed boost in confidence and the ability to face each day with renewed hope, resilience, and a stronger sense of self amidst this journey. The mutual support and camaraderie alleviate some of the burdens and provide a renewed sense of purpose and shared purpose in the face of the complex challenges presented by the disease. It is, in essence, an investment in your well-being and resilience, proving invaluable in the long and sometimes arduous journey of living with Alzheimer's disease. And for caregivers, this mutual support often translates into a renewed sense of being able to continue their caring journey with fresh strength and perspective.

7.5 Looking Ahead

The journey with Alzheimer's, while undeniably challenging, isn't solely defined by its difficulties. It's about embracing the present, cherishing the moments, and finding peace in the face of uncertainty. This doesn't negate the pain or the struggles; it acknowledges their presence while simultaneously highlighting the potential for profound growth, resilience, and unexpected joy. Focusing solely on the disease itself risks overshadowing the richness of life that continues to exist, even amidst the cognitive decline. Remember the person, not just the diagnosis. Remember their laughter, their passions, their love.

For caregivers, looking ahead involves self-care. It's not selfish; it's essential. Burnout is a real threat, and prioritizing your own physical and mental health is not a luxury, but a necessity. Seek support groups, utilize respite care when available, and find activities that bring you joy and rejuvenation. Remember, you can't pour from an empty cup. Replenishing yourself allows you to give more effectively and compassionately to your loved one. Explore mindfulness techniques, engage in regular exercise, and connect with friends and family. Your well-being is inextricably linked to the well-being of the person you care for.

Looking ahead also means planning. Financial planning, legal documentation—these are crucial steps that should be taken early on. Understand the financial implications of long-term care, explore long-term care insurance options, and ensure legal documents, such as power of attorney and advance directives, are in place. This proactive approach will alleviate stress later and ensure your loved one's wishes are respected. Seek professional advice from financial planners and estate lawyers to navigate this often complex process. Don't hesitate to ask for help; many resources are available to guide you.

For those living with Alzheimer's, the future may feel uncertain. Focus on what you can control. Engage in activities you enjoy, even if they require modifications. Maintain social connections, even if it's just a short visit with a loved one. Find comfort in routines and familiar surroundings. These small moments of joy and connection can significantly impact your quality of life. Embrace the present moment, finding beauty and meaning in the everyday experiences, regardless of memory lapses or cognitive decline. Engage in reminiscing about cherished memories, sharing stories and photos with loved ones to foster a sense of continuity and belonging.

Furthermore, looking ahead involves acceptance. This doesn't mean giving up or resigning oneself to defeat. It signifies acknowledging the realities of the disease while simultaneously focusing on finding meaning and purpose in the present moment. Acceptance paves the way for finding joy in the simple things—a warm embrace, a shared meal, a moment of connection. Acceptance allows for a shift in perspective, enabling a deeper appreciation for the preciousness of life and relationships. It's about finding peace and understanding, not about resignation. It's a journey of continuous adaptation and acceptance of the changing circumstances.

Finally, remember that hope persists, even in the face of adversity. Hope is not the belief that everything will be alright, but the courage to face whatever may come, knowing you're not alone. Support groups provide invaluable opportunities to connect with others navigating similar journeys, sharing experiences, and offering mutual support and understanding. They offer a sense of community and validation, reminding you that you are not alone in your journey. Lean on those around you, accept assistance when offered, and celebrate the small victories along the way. The future may be uncertain, but it's not without hope. The power of connection, resilience, and acceptance can illuminate the path forward, one step at a time.

www.ingramcontent.com/pod-product-compliance
Lightning Source LLC
LaVergne TN
LVHW022012200926
848481LV00007B/2357
* 9 7 9 8 3 4 8 5 8 5 1 3 6 *